INNOILVATION

The Science of Producing Powerful and Safe Essential Oils

Dr. Doug Corrigan

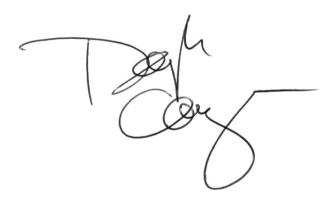

Doug Corrigan
Visit my website at www.StarFishScents.com

Printed in the United States of America

First Printing: Jan 2018
StarFishScents

ISBN-13 978-1983484704

"Understanding the science behind complex topics is one thing, but being able to teach it AND in a manner that is understandable is another thing all together. In 'Innoilvation', Mr. Corrigan has done a fantastic job of breaking down the science behind essential oils, their purity and the testing procedures utilized in the industry. A must read for every person using oils and wanting to ensure they are using the best quality products for their family"

–Dr. Jim Bob Haggerton, Doctor of Chiropractic Medicine and Founder of Essential Oil Club

"If you are at all interested in safely using essential oils as part of your wellness protocol, this book is a must read! In layman's terms, Dr. Doug Corrigan introduces you to the world of essential oils – where they come from, how they are grown, and most importantly, how they are tested. Know your essential oil provider – be a knowledgeable consumer – read this book!"

–James McDonald, Crown Diamond, Young Living

Look deep into nature, and then you will understand everything better.

—ALBERT EINSTEIN

About the Author

Dr. Doug Corrigan was led into the world of essential oils by his beautiful but persistent wife, Amy. That first kit was purchased for his wife to keep her from burning down the house with candles, but it eventually transformed their entire family and lifestyle.

Doug has a Ph.D. in Biochemistry and Molecular Biology, a Masters in Physics (concentration in Materials Science), and a Bachelors in Physics with a minor in Electrical Engineering. He started out in his career working for NASA on a series of microgravity research studies that flew aboard the Space Shuttle, as well as the Department of Energy doing research on new advanced materials. He then switched into the life sciences and launched a biotechnology company that developed novel molecular biology tools to help large pharmaceutical companies discover new drugs faster and more accurately. He is also an avid inventor, and has won over 30 different awards and licenses for his innovations that span from biotech, to nanoscience, to medicine, to energy technologies.

After witnessing the incredible benefits of essential oils being used on his family, Doug had to readapt his entire westernized school of thought to understand the science underlying essential oils. Through his studies, he realized that there is a "theory gap" between western science and natural medicine, and so he developed a model to connect these two disparate worlds. He now uses this model to teach in-depth online video classes that walk a person with no background in science through the basics of biochemistry, molecular biology, and how they relate ultimately to the science of essential oils.

Doug lives in North Carolina with his four wonderful children and his wife, Amy. He has a son who is basically a clone of himself, and three daughters. In his spare time, Doug loves to compose music on the piano and has published four albums: Fingers, Baby Fingers, Fingers Vol. II, and Drops of Rain (an album specifically created for relaxation and aromatherapy).

You can contact Doug with any questions by emailing
DrDougOilScience@gmail.com

You can find more educational content developed by Dr. Doug Corrigan about the science of essential oils at:

www.StarFishScents.com

Acknowledgements

I want to thank by wife, Amy – who has always encouraged me to follow my dreams and to reach for the stars. It's because of her that our family has found the wonderful health benefits of using essential oils. Without her, our family would fall apart, the earth would stop spinning, and the space-time continuum would rupture and peel apart into ten-gazillion fragments of chaotic madness, leaving us all destitute and naked for the eons to come.

CONTENTS

PREFACE

Are you thinking about starting down the road of using essential oils? With the hundreds of different choices that are now available, are you confused about what factors you should consider to ensure that the oils you use on you and your family are safe, pure, and effective? Is there a way to measure quality that's consistent and thorough? What is the science of the different quality control methods that should be used to ensure oil quality and safety, and how can a non-scientist hope to understand these methods? What qualities and scientific standards should you look for in an essential oil company?

These questions are what motivated me to write this booklet. Your time is valuable, so this booklet is short and to the point.

My hope is it will help you to answer these questions to ease your own mind, and will shed light on some of the science that goes into essential oils. Although my Ph.D. is in Biochemistry and Molecular Biology, this book is written for the non-scientist. In less than 50 pages, I anticipate that you will understand a great deal more about the complex factors that go into producing an essential oil that is therapeutically active, while maintaining safety and consistency. Perhaps you're already an avid user of essential oils and these considerations never came across your journey. This book is for you, too! I'm certain that you will learn something valuable that you can share with others.

At the end of the book, there is a checklist that you can use to evaluate the quality control standards of different essential oil companies to help you in your decision process. I hope that this tool is helpful to you and the friends, family, and colleagues in your life.

I. WHERE DO I START?

General Considerations for Choosing an Essential Oil Company

I f you already use essential oils, or are thinking about getting started with essential oils, it's very important to realize that your health depends on the make-up of the essential oil that you are introducing into your body through inhalation, topical application, or ingestion. When you use an essential oil, the molecules are readily transported into your systemic blood circulation, and then to the different organs and tissues in your body. Depending on the quality, purity, and composition of the essential oil, these molecules can either do you harm, provide you with no health benefit whatsoever, or provide you with incredible health benefits.

The purpose of this booklet is to educate people about what factors control the chemistry of essential oils, and the analytical techniques that are used to verify an oil's authenticity, purity, bioactivity, and safety. If your oil has any of the following components, your health could be compromised:

1) Adulterants – bad!

2) Synthetics – bad!

3) Solvents – bad!

4) Pesticides – bad!

5) Plasticizers – bad!

6) Heavy Metals – bad!

7) Other organic and inorganic impurities – bad!

8) Improper ratio of the naturally occurring components– Not dangerous, but certainly not helpful!

9) Natural components that are "missing" from the oil, especially trace components that account for the "synergy" of the oil– Again, not dangerous, but not efficacious, either.

It's very important to understand that just because an oil is free of adulterants and impurities, that does not guarantee that the oil will work therapeutically. The oil could easily be missing certain constituents that are necessary for the oil's therapeutic effect. The constituents may only be present in the oil if the plant was grown with the correct seed chemotype, soil conditions, harvesting conditions, and distillation process (discussed in more detail later).

Essential oils are complex mixtures of many different chemical compounds (each compound referred to as a "constituent"). Essential oils are never made of a singular chemical compound and, therefore, it is very difficult to comprehensively uncover an oil's complete constituent profile. Every oil is different, but the number of constituents in a particular oil may range from somewhere close to 20 constituents, all the way up to approximately 300 constituents!

How is it possible to consistently produce an oil with hundreds of constituents in the proper ratios, and verify that they are all there? How is it possible to verify that the source of the constituents are from a natural plant, and not synthetically produced in a laboratory (This is extremely challenging, and requires sophisticated equipment)? How is it possible to ascertain if an oil has been adulterated with solvents, oils, or other chemicals that may be hazardous to your health? This booklet will help you understand the answer these questions.

Many people have learned a hard lesson from this chilling fact: there are plenty of essential oil companies that are not properly labeling their oils. They are not being truthful with the contents inside the bottle. In many circumstances, these companies have absolutely no clue about the chemical composition of the oil because they didn't run the right set of tests on the oil. There are countless documented cases of oils being adulterated with harmful chemicals, even though the bottle is labeled natural. Manufacturers are more than likely not going to reveal to you if an oil contains plasticizers, heavy metals, or pesticides. In fact, in many cases they do not know this information because the oil was never tested and it was acquired from other unverified sources.

Some components are present in very small concentrations (trace components), and may not be measured by many instruments if particular techniques are not used. Therefore, an oil may show 20 constituents when using one analytical technique, but when a more rigorous set of techniques and procedures are used, 300 different constituents may make themselves known. Some trace components may only be present in a concentration of less than 0.1 %, but their presence is necessary to impart the correct therapeutic bioactivity of the oil through synergistic interactions in the cell. Therefore, it is important to use analytical techniques that possess the capability to accurately and reliably identify compounds that occur at minute concentrations.

This is an important lesson to learn: There is not one analytical technique that will reveal every component in an oil. There are many companies that tell you that they run Gas Chromatography – Mass Spectrometry (GC/MS) on their oils, but this is only one piece of the puzzle. GC/MS can only tell you so much, and if the proper techniques, columns, parameters, and libraries are not being used, the information is unreliable and deficient.

It's just as important to know what is in an oil as it is to know what is NOT in an oil. I'm going to repeat that statement, because I think it is one of the most important lessons to learn about assessing the quality and safety of an oil:

> *It's just as important to know what is in an oil as it is to know what is NOT in an oil.*

It is considerably more difficult to identify what is NOT in an oil. It is also very difficult to exhaustively and conclusively identify everything that IS in an oil. In order to do both, many different analytical techniques applied collectively are necessary to fully expose the vast array of different molecules that are present (and absent) in an oil.

When choosing an essential oil company, the first thing you should do is verify if they have an advanced laboratory (that they own and operate) that is filled with the equipment listed in this booklet, and that is staffed with scientists and technicians that have many years of specific experience with analyzing essential oils. If they are outsourcing this, or if they are only performing one or two of these tests, or none of these tests, then cross them off your list. Your family's health and safety are too important to even consider these companies. And there are many companies that fit into this cross-off-your-list category, and new ones are popping up each day.

In addition to owning and operating an advanced laboratory with the proper repertoire of analytical equipment, the lab should also possess an extensive library for proper identification of the thousands of different molecules that are found as components in essential oils. Without the proper software and chemical libraries, it is impossible to identify many of the components that are found in essential oils, especially some of the less common constituents (and derivatives) that are not routinely found in the standard commercial libraries. These libraries are internally augmented and advanced over time and, therefore, companies that have been conducting essential oil analysis the longest will tend to have the most comprehensive libraries that are specific to essential oils.

For this reason, one important criteria to consider is how long the company has been involved in the science and art of essential oils. It's important to identify a company that has been developing internal processes, standards, libraries, and techniques for a substantial amount of time. In the world of essential oil science:

Time =

    Experience =

        Knowledge =

            Quality, Safety, and Efficacy

There is no substitution for time and experience. There are no short cuts. You will soon see why after you have finished reading this booklet.

Another major factor to consider is the entire chain of events from when the seed enters the ground, to the time it is harvested, to the time it is distilled, to the time it is analyzed and sealed in a bottle for shipping to the consumer. How does the essential oil company control, monitor, and audit the entire lifecycle of this process? Do they have a comprehensive quality control process in place, and what portion of the entire process does this quality control process apply to? In other words, does their process control the entire chain of events from the beginning (seed going in the ground) to the end (bottle being sealed) that ensures the oils are consistent from batch to batch? Are batches not meeting the standard rejected without compromise?

Does the company ensure that the soil used to grow the plants is free of pesticides, pollutants, and heavy metals? Do they use a cultivation practice that is free of toxic pesticides and herbicides? Do they have distillation equipment that is free of plastic materials to ensure that plasticizers are not being introduced into the oil? Many studies have been published on the rampant contamination of essential oils with plasticizers and pesticides.

As you will learn in the next section, the composition of the oil is intimately connected to the type of seed, the soil conditions, the growth conditions, harvesting time and process, distillation process, as well as many other factors. A vital question for the company under consideration is if they own the process from beginning to end? Do they own their own farms? How many farms do they own, and are these farms globally distributed in such a way to produce oils with optimal composition? Do they perform the distillation process? If they partner with other farms, do they make that farm follow their quality control process, certify them, and audit them? Does the company even have the in-depth, experiential knowledge to create a process that others can adhere to, or do they simply rely on their suppliers to work it out for themselves?

Another major consideration is the history of the company and how their story directly connects to the long history of essential oil science. When you choose an essential oil company, you should ask, who started the company? Who did they train under? Where did they gain their knowledge? How many years of experience do they have specifically with understanding the science of essential oils? Did they just recently get into the business on a whim? Have they ever farmed the plants, and conducted the distillation process to gain an understanding of the complexity of essential oils? Or, did they just decide to start selling essential oils by purchasing them from other sources?

The medical understanding of essential oils and plant extracts extends back thousands of years. The Chinese, Egyptians, Indians, Grecians, Romans, Persians, etc, have all documented the therapeutic use of plant extracts in multiple ancient manuscripts. This knowledge was not translated into the modern era until scientists, doctors, and chemists in France began formalizing and advancing this knowledge in the practice of "aromatherapy" in the 19th and 20th centuries. These "fathers of aromatherapy" include individuals such as René-Maurice Gattefossé, Jean Valnet, Paul Belaiche, Jean-Claude Lapraz, Daniel Pénoël, and Pierre Franchomme. During the 1800's and 1900's, these pioneers reinvigorated the ancient use of essential oils and plant extracts, and reframed their use into what is now known as aromatherapy.

In terms of choosing an essential oil company, it's important to pay attention to the connection between the founders of the company and learning the science of growing, harvesting, and distilling essential oils from these experts. How is the company tied to this important historical body of knowledge that has preceded them? This knowledge is not readily available on every street corner, and it is almost impossible to learn simply by reading a book.

How does the company conduct business? Do they have a system of values in place that enables them to be good stewards over the earth and to conduct business responsibly and ethically? Does the company source their oils sustainably? Do they uplift the economy and infrastructure of local communities, and do they go above and beyond to comply with local environmental rules? Do they have a program in place that defines standards to protect delicate landscapes, plants, and wildlife? Do these standards include parameters for knowing where, how, and how much to plant and harvest, and the process used to reforest harvested trees?

These are some of the general questions you should first ask when choosing an essential oil. It seems like common sense, right?

To sum up, these are some important questions to consider when choosing an essential oil company (see the checklist at the end of the book for more detail):

1) Does the company own and operate an advanced analytical laboratory that is filled with the equipment listed in this booklet?

2) Is this lab staffed with scientists and technicians that possess specific experience analyzing essential oils? How many years of combined experience (specific to the analysis of essential oils) do they have?

3) Does this lab possess a comprehensive chemical and software library that is built up over time and that is specific to analyzing the thousands of constituents (and their derivatives) found in essential oils?

4) Does the lab routinely check for pesticides, plasticizers, heavy metals, adulterants, synthetics, solvents, and other harmful contaminants? Also, does the company have processes in place to ensure that pesticides, herbicides, and plasticizers are not being introduced into the oil during the growth and distillation process? (Remember: It's just as important to know what is in an oil as it is to know what is NOT in an oil.)

5) Does the lab use sophisticated enough techniques, libraries, and scientists that can analyze the oil for both major and minor (trace) constituents, to ensure that they are ALL present in their proper ratios and limits to provide the proper therapeutic efficacy?

6) What is the history of the company and its founders? How long have they been in operation, and what is the specific experience of the core team? Do they have extensive experience with the art and science of growing, harvesting, distilling, and performing quality control analysis on essential oils?

7) Does the company and its founders connect to the long history of essential oil science and knowledge through the "fathers of aromatherapy" that preceded them?

8) Does the company have an extensive quality control process that begins with the seed entering the ground, and that covers the entire chain of events that lead to the production and validation of the essential oil that's sealed in the bottle? Does this quality control

program ensure that oils are consistent from batch to batch, and that the oils not meeting these standards are rejected?

9) Does the company own its own farms and distilleries-- and if it partners with other farms-- does it ensure that those partners abide by the same practices and verify this through certification, auditing and inspection?

10) How does the company conduct business? Does the company have a stewardship and sustainability program in place to ensure that they are growing plants according to local and national regulations, and are they ensuring that they are practicing ecological practices that are sustainable and that protect the environment?

To take this discussion a bit further, in the following pages you will learn about the major factors that control the final composition of an essential oil. You will also learn about the different analytical techniques used to measure the composition of an essential oil and to ensure proper quality control specifications are met that are tied to safety and efficacy. You will learn how these techniques work and why they are important. If you don't have science background, do not worry! I purposefully made this booklet so that it is understandable to the non-scientist.

II. WHAT CONTROLS ESSENTIAL OIL QUALITY?

Factors that Determine the Composition of an Essential Oil

Many variables control the final composition of the oil. In fact, most people do not fully appreciate how complex the connection is between the entire process used to create the oil and the final constituent profile. The therapeutic potential of the oil starts with the seed and the composition of the soil that is used to cultivate the plant. The techniques used to cultivate the plant and to harvest the plant can dramatically influence the final chemical composition of the oil. After harvesting, the parameters used to control the extraction process are crucial to producing the correct composition profile of the final oil. After production, the right set of analytical techniques, instrumentation, and trained professionals are required to measure the composition, quality, and purity of the essential oil. It's vital that a company uses a quality control standard that governs this entire chain of events from the time the seed goes into the ground, to the time the oil is bottled.

The purpose of this booklet is not to go into too much detail regarding each of these factors, but to give you an overview that provides you with an appreciation of the process. If you're interested in learning specifics of how each of these factors control the composition of the oil, I have other educational resources available on www.StarFishScents.com that go into more detail.

Briefly, the variables that greatly impact the final composition of the oil include:

1) Chemotype of the Seed - Simply specifying the species of plant is not enough. There are subtypes of each plant species which vary based on the previous cultivation and reproduction history of the plant, and these are referred to as "chemotypes." The chemotype of the seed can drastically alter the final essential oil composition. Certain constituents can be present, or absent, or in drastically different ratios compared to other chemotypes from the same species. Therefore, to end up with consistent composition of oil, it's imperative that the same seed chemotype is used each time a new crop is produced. There can be 6 or more different chemotype varieties for each plant species, so simply paying attention to the species is not sufficient. If the essential oil company you are evaluating is not involved with the process from the time the seed goes in the ground, it is highly probable that they aren't paying attention to the seed chemotype, and there is a good possibility that they don't have access to this level of information. This is especially true of companies that simply purchase their supply of oils through brokers.

2) Soil Conditions – This includes factors such as nutrient profile, bacteria and other organisms living in the soil, soil moisture, soil pH, and soil aeration. Many of these soil factors are controlled by cultivation practices. It is much easier for soil conditions to be developed and perfected if the company has access to their own farms.

3) Geography and Environmental Conditions – Geography plays into things like relative humidity throughout the year, soil conditions, amount of rain fall, solar exposure throughout the growing cycle, etc. These factors are important to controlling the final composition of the essential oil.

4) Cultivation Practices – Factors such as: how the soil is tilled; how the seeds are planted; the types of fertilizers that are used on the plants; and the methods used to control the growth of weeds and the warding off of pests, are all critical to controlling the final composition of the oil. Ownership and control of farms enables a company to perfect proprietary growing practices that are tied to optimizing the therapeutic quality of the final oil.

5) Harvesting – The time of year, the time of month, and the time of day that the plant biomass is harvested all play a substantial role in producing the final chemistry of the oil. The presence or absence of certain constituents change throughout the growing cycle, and in some species of plants, dramatic changes can be seen over a 24-hour period. In addition, the part of the plant that is used (flower, petal, stem, wood, bark, leaf, root, etc) dictates the final composition of the oil. The ratio of left- and right-handed forms of certain molecules ("enantiomers", discussed in more detail below) in an essential oil can change throughout the growing cycle, altering the therapeutic activity of the oil. Ideally, an essential oil company should have processes in place to use the optimal part of the plant, and to harvest the plant at the correct time of year, time of month, and time of day. The company should understand the correlation of those variables with the final quality standard of the oil, and control for them in their process.

6) Distillation Process – Distillation is one of the major processes used to extract the essential oil constituents from the plant. The biomass of the plant is placed in a pressure vessel, and hot steam or water is used to extract the volatile components out of the plant tissue. Through a cooling process, this hot steam and essential oil mixture is converted back into a liquid form, and the essential oils are mechanically separated from the water fraction (In general, essential oils and water do not mix). It has been shown that the temperature, pressure, and time of this distillation process greatly affects the final composition of the oil. If you distill for too long, the molecules will be destroyed through thermal inactivation and oxidation. If you do not distill long enough, the minor constituents (trace components) will be missing from the oil. To produce an oil that is comprised of molecules (major and minor/trace) in the proper proportions that are not thermally degraded, the right time, pressure, and temperature profile must be used. Ownership and control of distillation facilities enables a company to develop and optimize this process for each oil. Ideally, each oil requires a different set of distillation conditions which are optimized for the compositional profile of that particular oil.

Another very important factor to consider is the materials that are in use in the distillation apparatus. Any plastic components in the entire chain of the distillation apparatus will liberate hazardous plasticizers into the essential oils. Plasticizers are routinely found in many of the essential oils that are available in the open market, simply because plastic materials were used either in the distillation equipment, or the handling containers. Essential oils are very efficient at extracting and dissolving plasticizers from plastics, and all plasticizers have been shown to be hazardous to our health, even in small quantities. Plastics are widely used in distillation equipment because they are much cheaper than stainless steel and glass.

7) Quality Control Process– After the distillation of the oil, the analytical techniques that are used to verify the composition of the oil are imperative. The entire chain of events that lead up to bottling of the oil is quite complex, and small variations in that entire chain can lead to changes in the oil composition. Therefore, a strict, defined, and thorough quality control process is needed in order to validate the presence (and absence) of certain chemical species in the final oil. Only after these quality control checks are completed, can the oil be released to the consumer.

The ideal essential oil company will address and control each of the 7 factors listed above. Many oil companies simply buy their oils on the open market from third-parties and, as a result, they cannot fully validate the first 6 factors that were used to produce that oil. They may, for example, have just purchased a lot of essential oil labeled "Lavender," but they have no inclination as to the composition of the oil because they weren't involved in how the oil was produced from start to finish. Therefore, they are left with the robustness of their quality control process to fully understand what is in the oil (and not in the oil). If you're not familiar with the exact process of how the oil was produced from start to finish, it is very difficult to ascertain the complete essential oil composition. As you will learn below, the analytical techniques that are currently used to understand the chemistry of essential oils can only tell you so much.

Many of these companies only run a GC/MS (discussed below) on the oil, and use that as their sole validation that the oil is ok to send to the consumer. As will be seen, a GC/MS can only tell you a limited amount of information about the oil. Depending on the techniques, libraries, and instrumentation used to perform the GC/MS, the presence of pesticides, plasticizers, and heavy metals will not be elucidated. Also, the presence of synthetics and impurities may not be evident. In addition, left and right-handed forms of certain molecules may not be differentiated (discussed below), and the presence of trace components will not be identified.

Therefore, other techniques are needed to form a complete picture, and many of the essential oil companies are not performing these other techniques. When you realize that these other companies use an inadequate or overly simplistic quality control process, along with fact that they have no control or oversight of the seed, cultivation, harvesting, or distillation process, it's easy to picture how these oils could be either hazardous or inconsequential to your health.

III. HOW SHOULD OILS BE ANALYZED?

The Analytical Techniques Necessary to Validate the Quality and Safety of an Essential Oil

GAS CHROMATOGRAPHY/MASS SPECTROMETRY(GC/MS)

The workhorse of analytical techniques for identifying the constituents in essential oils is GC/MS. I will describe basically how this instrument works, what it can tell you, and what it can't tell you. After you appreciate the entire set of factors that are necessary to achieve a successful GC/MS of an essential oil, it will become obvious that not just any analytical lab can run a GC/MS of an essential oil and produce meaningful data that accurately describes the constituents in that oil. Proper instrumentation, parameters, calibration, libraries, and experienced professionals who understand the peculiarities and limitations associated with GC/MS of essential oils are all necessary to accurately identify the constituents in an essential oil.

Since essential oils are complex mixtures of dozens to hundreds of different molecules, these molecules need to be isolated from one another before each one can be analyzed to determine its identity. GC/MS is a two-step process:

> Step 1- Use Gas Chromatography to separate the molecules from one another.
> Step 2- Use Mass spectrometry to identify each molecule.

Let's discuss the separation process first. In general, when you hear the word "Chromatography," think of "separation." There are many different forms of chromatography that are used in chemistry and biochemistry, each having their own methodologies, drawbacks, and strengths. "Gas" Chromatography is a separation process that occurs after the molecules have been converted into the gas phase. Because essential oils consist mainly of volatile components (meaning that they enter the gas phase quite easily), Gas Chromatography is a perfect technique to separate many of the compounds found in the essential oil. In Gas Chromatography, the following process and considerations are important:

1) The liquid form of the essential oils is injected into the GC instrument using a syringe that measures a certain amount of the liquid.

2) The oils are heated to a certain temperature to accelerate their release into the gas phase.

3) The oil vapors are combined with a stream of an inert carrier gas, like Helium or Nitrogen, that helps dilute and carry the gaseous essential oil compounds into the long column that will separate the molecules.

4) The gaseous molecules enter a long column (i.e. a separation "tube") that is usually 30 meters – 60 meters in length. Because it is very long, it is coiled up in a circular geometry to conserve space. The column has an internal diameter that is very narrow that allows the gaseous molecules to travel through the opening in the tube.

5) As the molecules travel down the length of this tube in the gas phase, they interact with the internal surface of the tube. This internal surface is made from a special solid material that has a certain affinity for the different molecules in the gas phase. Some of the molecules are very attracted to this solid material and, therefore, travel down the tube at a slower rate. Some molecules are not very attracted to this solid material, and travel down the tube at a much faster rate. Because each molecule that makes up the essential oil is different, they each have a different affinity for the solid material that lines the column. As the molecules travel down the tube at a different speed, they will begin to separate from one another. There are many different solid materials that can be used, and each solid material separates the components in a complex mixture differently. Choosing the right solid material that optimizes the separation of essential oil molecules is critical. The diagram below demonstrates the principle of how the interaction of the inner wall and the molecules causes the different constituents to move at different speeds and separate from one another as they travel through the inner tube of the column.

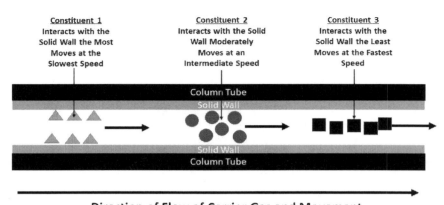

Direction of Flow of Carrier Gas and Movement
Through the Column

Figure 1 – Interaction of Different Constituents with the Solid Material Lining the Separation Tube of a Gas Chromatography Instrument

6) To make successful measurements on each molecule, they must be isolated/separated from one another. The major factors that ultimately control how well the molecules separate from one another are:

- The length of the column
- The inner diameter of the column
- The inlet temperature that is used to vaporize the liquid sample into the gas phase
- The temperature at which the column is maintained. If the temperature is changed throughout the separation process, then an additional factor to be considered is the rate of change of this temperature
- The type of carrier gas and its rate of flow
- The type of solid material lining the column
- The thickness of the solid material lining the column

Each of these factors need to be optimized to effectively separate the molecules that make up a particular essential oil. If one set of parameters is used to separate a certain type of chemistry, it doesn't necessarily mean that these same parameters can be used to separate an essential oil. In fact, if one set of parameters is optimized to separate the components of Lavender, it doesn't mean that the same set of parameters can be used to optimally separate the components of Frankincense. These parameters need to be tweaked based on the chemistry of the mixture to be separated. Again, it is evident that many years of essential-oil specific training are needed for lab technicians and analysts who perform GC/MS on essential oils. If a technician has years of experience running and interpreting a GC/MS in a pharmaceutical lab, for example, this is not sufficient training to allow this person to begin running and interpreting GC/MS for essential oils. This person needs to train under a professional who has worked with essential oils for most of their career to understand the vast array of variables and considerations that need be accounted for.

7) Retention Time- If each of the factors listed above are precisely controlled, then each molecule will separate from the others and will exit the end of the column at a characteristic time, called the retention time. When the molecule exits the column, it will form a "peak" on the chromatogram, which is a plot of the concentration of molecules exiting the column over time. Each molecule in an essential oil can be defined by a specific Retention Index, which is unique to that chemical constituent. If different constituents interact similarly with the column, then they will have very similar retention indices, making it very difficult to resolve them through separation. Labs that have not optimized their columns and parameters will run into this problem of inadequate separation. In this scenario, instead of having one molecule in each

peak of the chromatogram, there may be several compounds in the same peak, making it very difficult to identify each of them. An optimized GC process will have each of the factors listed above fine-tuned to result in optimal separation. Retention times are one way to assign the identify of a molecule; however, it is certainly not a full proof method. Many molecules have such similar retention indices that it is near impossible to uniquely identify them by simply relying on their retention times. Also, depending on the resolution of the instrument and the process, it may be impossible to do this for certain compounds because they are not adequately separated from one another.

8) Mass Spectrometry - After the molecules leave the column, they are introduced into the mass spectrometer at the same time they exit the chromatography column for proper identification. Essentially, a mass spectrometer is an instrument that can measure the mass of an individual molecule. It can also break up the molecules into smaller pieces and measure the masses of those smaller pieces. The mass of the parent molecule, and the masses of the smaller fragmented pieces, create a mass "fingerprint" of the molecule. For the most part, each unique molecule has a unique mass fingerprint; however, this is not always true. Many molecules that are "similar" can provide the same mass fingerprint information, and therefore, false identities can be assigned. This is a problem with essential oil molecules because many of the different molecules in essential oils are very similar to one another and, therefore, provide identical mass spectral fingerprints. This is especially true of molecules that are essentially mirror images of each other ("enantiomers"), which are discussed in more detail later.

When you combine the mass spectra data along with the retention index of the molecule, they go a very long way in terms of properly identifying a molecule. However, there are plenty of scenarios where a molecule can be falsely identified by the combination of retention index and mass spectra. Many molecules give very similar retention indices and mass fingerprints. This is especially true of isomers, and there are many isomers lurking in essential oil chemistry. Isomers are molecules that are identical in molecular weight but have a slightly different arrangement of atoms in the molecule. So, although GC/MS is a good first step to identify the presence of molecules in an essential oil, it is certainly not exhaustive, not without error, and ambiguity can rear its ugly head. Other techniques are needed to fully resolve the components that are present in an oil (and absent).

9) Library – There are two different types of libraries:

a) Software library – A GC/MS software library is a list of all the retention indices and mass fingerprints for each molecule. If the library is small, the instrument will not be able to identify most constituents. The larger the library, the greater the instrument's ability to identify a greater variety of constituents. A non-exhaustive library will lead to misidentifications (false positives and false negatives).

b) Chemical library – It's important to possess "standards" that can be run on the GC/MS instrument to calibrate the instrument. These standards can be the individual constituents, or the entire oil (previous batches that set a "standard" benchmark). A chemical library can be used as a benchmark to compare future batches of oils, and to ensure the instrument is running properly from run to run. Also, the chemical library can help to fill in gaps that the initial software library may have.

An important consideration in evaluating the merits of an essential oil company is the size and complexity of the software library and chemical library. Libraries are larger in size (and therefore more accurate in assigning identities to the molecules) for companies that are more mature. It requires time and running thousands to tens of thousands of samples to fully build out an extensive library. Most of the software libraries that GC instruments come equipped with are inadequate to identify the tens of thousands of different molecules (and their derivatives) that are present in different essential oils.

A center of excellence for establishing standards for essential oil composition and analysis is the Centre National de la Recherche Scientifique (National Center for Scientific Research) in France (CNRS). Dr. Herve Casabianca served as the chairman of the Committee of Essential Oil Standards for the Association Française de Normalisation Organization Regulation (AFNOR)/ International Standards Organization (ISO). AFNOR was created in 1926 as the hub for standards in France, and consists of nearly 2,500 member companies. Its aim is to lead and coordinate the standards development process and to promote the application of those standards. Dr. Casabianca is an expert on gas chromatography analysis and other important analytical techniques as they pertain to measuring and setting standards for essential oils, and he is intimately involved in AFNOR standards for essential oils.

Based on what you now know about GC/MS, you can now understand the following limitations inherent to GC/MS with respect to analyzing essential oils:

1) Depending on the resolving power of the column, the parameters being used during the run, and the library, certain constituents that are present will go unrecognized (false negative), and certain constituents that are not present will be identified (false positive). The rate of false positives and false negatives increase when the system is not optimized.

2) Certain constituents will not be identified that are present in a lower concentration than the lower detection limit of the instrument. This is related to the instrument's sensitivity.

3) It's very difficult to resolve left and right-handed forms of molecules (mirror images) with a normal GC/MS. Both forms of the molecule will exit the column at the same time, and both will give identical mass spectral fingerprints. This becomes a problem for identifying synthetic adulterants, because many synthetics have a different ratio of left to right handed forms of the molecule than the natural source. A special type of GC/MS, termed "chiral" GC/MS is needed to efficiently and accurately measure each component separately. Also, each form of the molecule has a completely different therapeutic profile. Therefore, it's important to measure the presence of one form of the molecule over the other to fully validate the therapeutic profile of an oil. A company that is paying attention to detail should use chiral GC/MS as a quality control measure in addition to normal GC/MS (discussed later).

4) A GC/MS can only measure molecules that readily evaporate when heated. Many constituents in essential oils have enough volatility to be measured on a GC/MS. This is especially true of lighter molecules. However, there are heavier, less volatile components in essential oils that are not easily measured in a gas

chromatograph. For these heavier molecules that are less volatile, a liquid chromatograph is required (discussed later). Also, some adulterants and impurities can only be effectively measured using liquid chromatography.

5) Heavy metals and other elements along the periodic table are not readily measured on a GC instrument. Other analytical techniques are required (discussed later).

6) To measure for the presence of plasticizers and pesticides (which are normally present in very low concentrations), very exotic modifications to the GC process (i.e., different preparation techniques to concentrate the pesticides and plasticizers, a different column, different parameters) are needed to specifically measure their presence. In addition, a GC may not have the ability to measure certain species if they are not volatile, and a liquid chromatography technique is needed.

This isn't a comprehensive list of the limitations of GC/MS, but it represents the major shortcomings. As you can see, GC/MS is not sufficient to verify every component that is, and isn't, in the oil. A collection of other techniques is necessary to fully elucidate the oil's composition. An important question to ask about any essential oil company is if they are running other tests in addition to GC/MS.

CHIRAL GAS CHROMATOGRAPHY

As mentioned above, many molecules can come in two different forms. These forms are "mirror images" of one another. The molecules possess the same chemical structure, but it's as if they were flipped in a mirror. To understand this better, your right and left hands are perfect examples of two structures that are mirror images of one another. Each hand has the same number of fingers, arranged and connected in the same way, but you can't directly overlay one on top of the other. However, if you take your right hand and reflect it in a mirror, it will perfectly overlap your left hand. Your right and left hands are mirror images. The picture below helps you to see this mirror-image property of your hands.

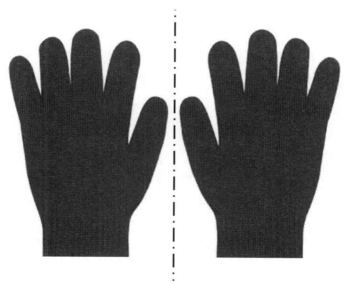

Figure 2 – Depiction of Left and Right-Handed Forms of Molecules Using Hands

The fancy name chemists give to molecules that are mirror images of one another is "enantiomers." Another term that is used to described them is "chiral." Chiral molecules are molecules that come in different right-handed and left-handed forms. Scientists give fancy names to simple concepts because it makes them sound smart.

Many of the constituents in an essential oil come in left and right-hand version. For example, let's discuss limonene, which is a common constituent found in many different essential oils. There are two forms of limonene: D-Limonene (the "right" handed version), and L-Limonene (the "left handed" version). D-Limonene is mostly found in citrus oils: orange, lemon, lime, etc. It has a distinct lemony smell. L-Limonene is found mostly in mint oils and has more of a piney smell to it.

Not only do D-Limonene and L-Limonene have completely different smells, they also work differently in your body. They have different bioactivity profiles.

Don't miss that last point because it's critical that you understand this concept. Even though chiral molecules have the same chemical formula and geometric arrangement of atoms, their activity is completely different. To your body, it's as if they are completely different molecules. Just like your right hand won't fit into a left-handed glove, neither will D-Limonene fit into the biological spaces that L-Limonene is designed to fit into, and vice versa.

Plants make different ratios of the two different forms of molecules, and this ratio can change throughout the growing cycle. In some instances, a plant will only make 100% of one form over the other. In other instances, it may be a 70%/30% mix of the two, and this ratio may change depending on the time of year and growing conditions. It really depends on the constituent and the plant itself.

When a constituent is artificially synthesized through a series of chemical reactions in the lab (rather than purifying it from its natural source), it is very difficult to synthesize one form over the other. Usually, chemical reactions that are performed in a lab or production facility produce an equal amount of the left and right-hand forms. It becomes quite a challenge to purify one away from the other. Let's say a plant normally makes 90% of the right form, and 10% of the left form a certain constituent. Now let's suppose that when you run on an analysis on the essential oil you find a 50%:50% mix of that constituent. That's a good indication that this oil has been "adulterated" with a synthetic version of the molecule.

Also, a common trick is to purify a constituent from a cheaper source and add it to a more expensive oil to make that oil cheaper per unit weight. In this case, the oil hasn't been adulterated by a synthetic version of a molecule, but by a natural form. If the cheaper plant produces that constituent in a different enantiomeric ratio than the more expensive oil, then measuring the ratio of the left-handed to right-handed versions of the molecule in the more expensive oil can be a method to determine if that oil has been adulterated.

Adulteration with synthetics and naturally produced constituents is a rampant problem with essential oils. There are many publications in the research literature that describe the pervasiveness of this problem and the difficulty this presents to analytical chemists to devise techniques that can measure when an oil has been adulterated. The tricksters have found ways to deceive the analytical instruments, especially GC/MS systems.

As described above in the section about GC/MS, a typical GC column does not separate the left-handed form of the molecule from the right-handed form. These two molecules come off the column at the same time in the same peak. And when these two molecules are simultaneously introduced into the mass spectrometer, they produce the exact same mass spectral fingerprint.

Is there an instrument that can easily differentiate these two forms accurately? Yes. A chiral GC instrument. How does it work?

The principals of chiral gas chromatography are the same as normal gas chromatography. A long column is used to separate the molecules from one another. The difference is in the solid material that lines the column. This material is specially chosen to interact with the left-handed form of the molecule differently than the right-handed form. In this way, the two different molecules travel down the tube at a different speed and become separated from one another.

So, why not use a chiral column for every GC test? The main reason is there isn't one solid material that can separate all chiral molecules equally. One particular chiral column may only be able to separate a small number of constituents. There isn't a "one-size-fits-all" chiral column, meaning that the analytical lab would need to be equipped with many different chiral columns to evaluate different constituents, and they would need to be prepared to make several different runs, which is very time consuming.

A chiral chromatography system should be a standard analytical capability of any company that sells essential oils; however, you will find that this is absolutely not the case. A chiral GC system is needed for two purposes:

1) Detecting certain forms of adulteration by synthetic or natural molecules.

2) Determining the therapeutic efficacy of the oil. Again, this is based on the fact that the right and left-handed forms of molecules act completely different in our bodies physiologically.

Because of the time, expense, and expertise that's needed to perform chiral GC analysis, most essential oil companies do not run this test. If an essential oil company doesn't perform chiral GC on their oils, this could easily translate into consumers unwittingly using adulterated oils and oils that lack the proper therapeutic profile.

HIGH PERFORMANCE LIQUID CHROMATOGRAPHY (HPLC)

Not all constituents in an essential oil are as volatile as others. The lighter weight components have a higher volatility and enter the gas phase readily to be separated in a gas chromatograph. However, oils with heavier, less volatile constituents cannot be fully evaluated using only a GC. This is especially true with essential oils that are derived from resinous sources, such as Frankincense and Myrrh. Therefore, a combination of GC and HPLC may be necessary to fully understand the complete list of constituents that are present in an oil. This is especially true for heavier weight components that may only be present in trace quantities.

This is where liquid chromatography is very useful. In liquid chromatography, the essential oil is not evaporated before introducing it into the separation column. Instead, the essential oil is maintained in the liquid form, and then introduced into the column for separation. Therefore, the constituents that are not volatile will be analyzed.

In addition, the presence of certain pesticides, plasticizers, and adulterating oils are more conducive to detection using liquid chromatography as opposed to gas chromatography.

The principals of liquid chromatography are essentially the same as was discussed in the section on GC. The type of column, length of column, type of solid material, etc. are all important factors to achieving a successful separation of the molecules. In High Performance Liquid Chromatography (HPLC), the liquid is pumped through the column at high pressure. The separation columns in an

HPLC instrument are much shorter than in a GC instrument, and the solid material that interacts with the molecules to separate them is configured differently. Other than that, the principles are the same. The molecules are separated from one another, and then identified using a mass spectrometer.

Again, the important factors that are necessary in achieving a successful run and analysis are:

1) Adjusting the parameters such that they are optimized for evaluating a particular essential oil.

2) Trained technicians and analysts that are experienced with the nuances associated with analyzing the complex chemistry presented by essential oils.

3) A vast software and sample library that is tailored to identifying the complex repertoire of molecules that are found in essential oils.

It's important to identify a company that performs liquid chromatography on their oils to ensure that certain contaminants and adulterants are absent from the oil, and to ensure that the oil possesses the full spectrum of constituents.

ISOTOPIC RATIO MASS SPECTROMETRY (IRMS)

IRMS is a very specialized, highly sophisticated analytical technique that is used, among other things, to measure whether the molecules that make up a given substance are natural or synthetic. Beyond this, IRMS is sensitive enough to identify the geographic location of the plant that was used to make the essential oil. This is probably the most difficult technique to understand, but I will do my best to make it easy.

To understand this technique and why it's important, it's first necessary to understand the definition of an isotope. Perhaps you are struggling to remember this term from high school chemistry, or perhaps you are a wizard at chemistry that has spent your career studying isotopes.

All molecules are just a combination of atoms that are connected into a specific shape. For example, water is a molecule that is made up of two hydrogen atoms connected to one oxygen atom. All of the available atoms that can be combined into different molecules are listed on the periodic table of the elements. There are over 100 different elements listed on this table, but only a handful of elements are present in the molecules that make up an essential oil. The top three elements that are found in essential oil molecules are: carbon, hydrogen, and oxygen. Very rarely is sulfur or nitrogen present.

Now, elements can be found in nature as different "isotopes". An isotope of an element has all of the same chemical properties as that element, but it has a different weight due to more or less neutrons residing in the nucleus of the atom. All atoms are made up of protons and neutrons (which reside in the central nucleus), and electrons (which are flying around in a cloud that surrounds the nucleus). The number of protons in the nucleus determines the name of the element. For example, carbon is defined as any atom that has 6 protons in the nucleus. Therefore, carbon is the 6th element that appears on the periodic table of the elements. Hydrogen is the first because it only has 1 proton in the nucleus. Oxygen is the eighth because it has 8 protons in the nucleus. The number of neutrons and electrons is irrelevant to naming the atom. The only factor that is considered when naming an atom is how many protons are in the nucleus.

Now, some atoms can exist in nature with a different number of neutrons residing in the nucleus. These make up the different "isotopes" of that atom. For example, the most abundant form of carbon found in nature is the isotope known as ^{12}C, which has 6 protons and 6 neutrons. Another isotope found in nature (but very rarely) is ^{13}C, which has 7 neutrons in the nucleus. Therefore, ^{13}C is heavier than ^{12}C. The same is true of Oxygen and hydrogen – they appear in nature as different isotopes.

What's important to understand is that the ratio of abundance of one isotope of an element found in nature to another isotope is relatively constant. So, if plants are taking in CO_2 from the atmosphere, they should be incorporating a certain ratio of ^{12}C and ^{13}C into their tissue and into the molecules that the plant produces from this carbon (the carbon atoms in essential oils are the same carbon atoms that the plant took in in the form of CO_2). Because a large fraction of the carbon in atmospheric CO_2 is found in the ^{12}C form (about 98.89%), and a tiny fraction of the Carbon in atmospheric CO_2 is found in the ^{13}C form (about 1.11%), the ratio of the different isotopes of carbon found in essential oils will be similar (but not exact– the reason for this is explained below).

Because ^{13}C is heavier than ^{12}C, plants do not incorporate the ^{13}C into their molecules as readily as the ^{12}C. Some plants incorporate it more readily than others, but never at the same ratio that is present in the atmosphere. Therefore, the ratio of ^{13}C to ^{12}C found in the molecules of plants is lower than the ratio of ^{13}C to ^{12}C found in the atmosphere. How much lower is based on the type of plant, and even the geography and environment in which it was grown. The same type of argument can be made for the isotopes of oxygen and the isotopes of hydrogen which make up essential oil molecules.

Therefore, the ratio of different isotopes found in the molecules of an essential oil can be an indicator of what type of plant produced the essential oil, and in some cases, where it was grown.

Effectively, this ratio of isotopes becomes a fingerprint that identifies the origin of the molecules.

Most synthetic chemicals are either derived from another plant, or from coal or petroleum. A large portion of the synthetic molecules which are used to adulterate essential oils are derived from petroleum. Coal and petroleum exhibit a considerably lower ^{13}C to ^{12}C ratio, and therefore any molecule that is synthesized in the lab from these sources will possess this same signature ratio of ^{13}C to ^{12}C. Therefore, IRMS can be used to fingerprint whether the molecules are naturally derived or synthetically derived. Also, if an oil has been adulterated by another oil or solvent, it will shift the overall ratio of isotopes, and this can be measured.

So, how does an IRMS work? The liquid sample is usually separated into its individual constituents using a GC. Then as each constituent exits the GC column it is combusted in the presence of oxygen at high temperature to produce CO_2 and H_2O. The H_2O is removed and the CO_2 is then sent to a very sophisticated mass spectrometer that can measure the amount of each carbon isotope that is present. From this, the ratio of ^{13}C to ^{12}C can be calculated. A similar method can be used to determine the ratio of oxygen or hydrogen isotopes.

IRMS instruments are very expensive and not routinely used. As you can see, this instrument is especially powerful for detecting adulteration and authenticity. This instrument should be a part of a company's toolkit; however, most companies are not utilizing this instrument's sensitivity and power because of the significant cost.

ORGANOLEPTIC TESTING

The power of the human nose is absolutely amazing. Humans have the capability to differentiate between millions of different odors, and to detect the presence of compounds that are present in concentrations less than 1 part per billion. The amazing network of olfactory receptors in our nasal cavity, combined with the olfactory bulb and olfactory cortex in our brain makes this complex detection process possible.

The ability to discriminate certain odors can be developed through years of training and experience. The organoleptic properties of a substance are those properties that can be readily differentiated through our senses: sight, touch, taste, and odor. Essential Oil Organoleptologists are individuals who have trained to recognize certain classes of odors with higher degrees of perception and discrimination than the average person. A highly trained organoleptologist who is an expert in essential oil odors can easily ascertain if too much or too little of an important constituent is present in an essential oil. An experienced organoleptologist can determine if an oil's overall profile is within range of the normal, and they can also tell very quickly if an oil has been adulterated with foreign contaminants. They may not be able to tell what it is exactly, but they will be able to say, "something just doesn't seem right."

What's the advantage of organoleptic testing with respect to the other techniques? First, it's very fast. An experienced organoleptologist can identify if a batch is generally within specification within seconds. Major problems are quickly identified. Organoleptic testing can be used for spot checking at different points along the production process. For example, organoleptic testing can be used to quickly screen at the site where the oils are being distilled to make sure the distillation process has proceeded correctly. In addition, highly trained organoleptologists can sometimes detect components that may not have been readily identifiable on one of the other instruments. Using this technique can serve as a good complement to the analytical techniques where human intuition and experience are more readily brought into the quality control process. This additional layer of testing serves as a great way to "double check" that the analytical instruments were correct in their assessment.

A reputable and experienced essential oil company should have staff members who have been working with essential oils for decades, and who are very familiar with the aroma profile of every oil in its most ideal state. Ideally, this experience should be developed by being involved in every step of the process. Companies that aren't involved with the growth, cultivation, harvesting, and distillation of the essential oil will have a much harder time developing this internal expertise simply because they don't have a baseline target to identify as the "standard." Since every batch they purchase is different, and correlations can't be made between seed chemotype, soil conditions, weather conditions, harvesting conditions, distillation conditions, and the aromatic profile of the oil, they are really shooting in the dark. Companies that control the entire process of producing an essential oil can consistently control the baseline and then train their organoleptologists to this baseline to detect deviations from the norm.

OTHER TECHNIQUES

There are other techniques which are very important to the quality control process should be used to paint a complete picture of the oil, and they are described briefly below:

Fourier Transform Infrared Spectroscopy (FTIR) – In this test, the samples are exposed to different wavelengths of infrared light, and the absorption of the light through the sample is measured at each wavelength. Certain chemicals or chemical "groups" absorb certain wavelengths more than others. Therefore, this absorption profile can be a "fingerprint" that helps to identify the presence of certain classes of molecules within the essential oil. This test can help to quickly uncover if the overall profile of the oils is within normal limits, and can sometimes be used to detect the presence of certain adulterants depending on their chemical identity. This test is a great spot check, but it is certainly not exhaustive enough to reveal the details about the composition of the oil.

Inductively Coupled Optical Emission Spectrometry (ICP–OES) and Inductively Coupled Plasma Mass Spectrometry (ICP–MS) – These analytical techniques subject the sample to a very high temperature in a flame, and then either measure the emission wavelengths of light given off by the different elements that are in the sample, or the mass of each element. The very nature of this technique breaks down the molecules into individual atoms and, therefore, it is impossible to determine the molecular composition of the sample using this technique. However, it can provide data on the presence of certain elements in the oil, such as heavy metals, minerals, and other contaminants. Heavy metal contamination in oils has been reported in the literature, and becomes more of a problem if the plants are grown near industrialized activity. Also, synthetics can possess high levels of heavy metals. Therefore, this type of test is crucial for validating that an oil is safe to use.

Refractometry (Refractive Index) – The refractive index is a measure of how fast light travels through the oil. The density of the oil and the overall chemical makeup determines how fast light travels through the oil. If an oil has the same chemistry as another oil, the refractive index should be the same. Therefore, this number serves as a quick way to initially determine if the oil is within limits. However, it is not conclusive. Two samples with the same refractive index do not necessarily have the same composition. It's a great spot check, but it is not definitive.

Specific Gravity – The specific gravity of an oil is a measure of its density. Most oils are less dense than water. If an oil is not made correctly, has a high water content, or is adulterated, its specific gravity can be different than the nominal. Like the other tests, this test is an appropriate method to perform a quick spot check, but it does not provide enough information to verify the complete composition of the oil.

Flash Point – The flash point is the minimum temperature of the oil that is necessary for the vapors to ignite when exposed to an ignition source. This temperature is a function of the overall composition of the oil. Adulterants, solvents, and water can dramatically impact the flash point temperature. Again, this an appropriate method to do a quick spot check, but it is not informative enough to provide any detail about the oil's chemical composition.

Peroxide Value – The peroxide value of an oil is a measure of the degree to which an oil has been oxidized. Essential oil compounds contain carbon-carbon double bonds, and these bonds can be oxidized in the presence of oxygen. This oxidation process naturally occurs in oils as they age, and this process is accelerated if the oils are subjected to air, light, and heat. As the oil becomes oxidized, it loses its therapeutic value. This instrument is used to ensure that every oil is fresh and has not been overly oxidized during the production process.

<u>Automated Micro-enumeration</u>- This instrument automatically counts if any microorganisms contaminate the sample, such as bacteria, yeast, or mold.

IV. CONCLUSION

What Have You Learned?

Now that you've finished reading this short booklet, I hope you have a much better understanding how complex essential oils are, and all of the factors that go into producing and analyzing the oils to ensure that they are safe and therapeutically active. Some people may argue that the considerations presented in this booklet are over extensive and unnecessary. To that person I would ask this question:

"How important is your health to you?"

Every single one of the factors and tests that I have outlined are necessary for ensuring the safety and the therapeutic potential of the essential oil. Remember,

> *It's just as important to know what is in an oil as it is to know what is NOT in an oil.*

The considerations presented in this book are designed to reveal what is in an oil, and what is not in an oil. Your health is too important to take shortcuts.

In the next section, there is a checklist that you can use to evaluate different essential oil companies that you may be considering or that you are already using.

V. CHECKLIST

*Checklist to Evaluate an Essential Oil
Company*

	Factor	Company 1	Company 2	Company 3	Company 4
Company	How Long has the Company Existed?				
	Who are the Founders?				
	Number of Years of Experience of the Founders				
	Are Founders Connected to Long History of Essential Oils?				
	Who Did The Founders Learn Essential Oil Science From?				
	Do They Produce Their Own Oils, Or Do They Simply Purchase, Bottle, and Resell?				
Analytical Laboratory	Do they Own an Operate an Analytical Lab, or is outsourced? Outsourced to who?				
	Number of Years of Combined Experience of the Technicians				
	Size of Library				
	GC/MS?				
	Chiral GC?				
	HPLC?				
	IRMS?				
	Organoleptic Testing?				
	FTIR?				
	ICP-OES/ICP-MS?				
	Refractometry?				
	Specific Gravity?				
	Flash Point?				
	Peroxide Value?				
	Automated Microenumeration?				
	Other Tests?				
	Is Testing Connected to any International Standards?				
	Does Quality Control Process Ensure Oils Not Meeting Standards are Rejected?				
Sourcing	Do They Own Their Own Farms?				
	How Many Farms Do they Own?				
	Where are the Farms Located?				
	Are pesticides used on the farms?				
	Do They Partner with Farms and Suppliers?				
	Do they Certify the Partners?				
	How Do They Certify the Partners?				
	Does Their Process Control the Seed, Cultivation, Growth, and Harvesting of the Plant?				
	Do they Conduct Audits/Inspections of the Farms to Ensure Compliance to Their Standards?				
	Do They Own Their Own Distillaries?				
	How Many Years of Experience with Distillation?				
	Are Plastic Materials Used in Their Distillation or Handling Equipment?				
	Do they have a Compliance and Sustainability Program?				

For a larger version to print, please visit www.StarFishScents.com

	Factor	Company 5	Company 6	Company 7	Company 8
Company	How Long has the Company Existed?				
	Who are the Founders?				
	Number of Years of Experience of the Founders				
	Are Founders Connected to Long History of Essential Oils?				
	Who Did The Founders Learn Essential Oil Science From?				
	Do They Produce Their Own Oils, Or Do They Simply Purchase, Bottle, and Resell?				
Analytical Laboratory	Do they Own an Operate an Analytical Lab, or is outsourced? Outsourced to who?				
	Number of Years of Combined Experience of the Technicians				
	Size of Library				
	GC/MS?				
	Chiral GC?				
	HPLC?				
	IRMS?				
	Organoleptic Testing?				
	FTIR?				
	ICP-OES/ICP-MS?				
	Refractometry?				
	Specific Gravity?				
	Flash Point?				
	Peroxide Value?				
	Automated Microenumeration?				
	Other Tests?				
	Is Testing Connected to any International Standards?				
	Does Quality Control Process Ensure Oils Not Meeting Standards are Rejected?				
Sourcing	Do They Own Their Own Farms?				
	How Many Farms Do they Own?				
	Where are the Farms Located?				
	Are pesticides used on the farms?				
	Do They Partner with Farms and Suppliers?				
	Do they Certify the Partners?				
	How Do They Certify the Partners?				
	Does Their Process Control the Seed, Cultivation, Growth, and Harvesting of the Plant?				
	Do they Conduct Audits/Inspections of the Farms to Ensure Compliance to Their Standards?				
	Do They Own Their Own Distillaries?				
	How Many Years of Experience with Distillation?				
	Are Plastic Materials Used in Their Distillation or Handling Equipment?				
	Do they have a Compliance and Sustainability Program?				

For a larger version to print, please visit www.StarFishScents.com

NOTES